BEYOND SWEAT AND TEARS.

How To Acquire the Body and Mind you desire with the help of Bio-hackers.

BONUS:30-Days Success Challenge:Your Practical Recipe For A Healthier You.

BY

Catherine. J. Norris

1

Beyond sweat and tears

Copyright

provided by [Catherine.J.Norris] and while we strive to keep the information up to date and correct, we make no representations or warranties of any kind, express or implied, about the completeness, accuracy, reliability, suitability, or availability concerning the information, products, services, or related graphics contained in [Beyond Sweat and Tears] for any purpose. Any reliance you place on such information is, therefore, strictly at your own risk.

In no event will we be liable for any loss or damage, including without limitation, indirect or consequential loss or damage, or any loss or damage whatsoever arising from loss of data or profits arising out of, or in connection with, the use of this book[Beyond Sweat and Tears].

Through this book [Beyond Sweat and Tears], you may be able to link to other websites that are not under the control of [Catherine.J.Norris]. We have no control over the nature, content, and availability of those sites. The inclusion of any links does not necessarily imply a recommendation or endorse the views expressed within them.

Every effort is made to keep [this book, website, or other content format] up and running smoothly. However, [Catherine.J.Norris] takes no responsibility for, and will not be liable for, [this book, website, or other content format] being temporarily unavailable due to technical issues beyond our control.

5

Beyond sweat and tears

About the Author

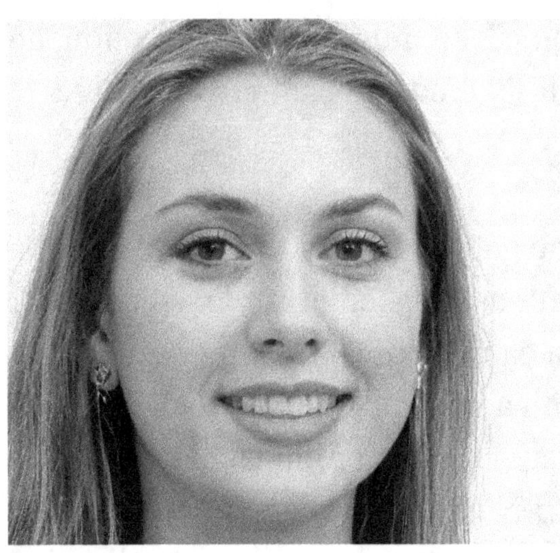

Meet Catherine.J.Norris, the visionary
force behind the pages you're about to explore.
A relentless explorer of the realms of health and
vitality, Catherine.J.Norris is not just an author
but a biohacking architect with a passion for
sculpting lives of wellness.

With an insatiable curiosity and a background in
Diet, weightloss, Catherine.J.Norris seamlessly
blends the art of scientific inquiry with the
poetry of holistic well-being. Embarking on a

mission to decode the secrets of vitality, Catherine.J.Norris weaves together the threads of nutrition, sleep, mind-body connection, and more, inviting readers on a transformative odyssey.

Beyond the pages, Catherine.J.Norris is a fervent advocate for a balanced lifestyle, where each day becomes a canvas for cultivating health and joy. Armed with a pen and a fervent belief in the transformative power of biohacking, Catherine.J.Norris invites you to join the journey—a journey where vibrant well-being is not just a destination but a way of life.

Get ready to explore, evolve, and embrace the full spectrum of vitality as guided by the architect of well-being, Catherine.J.Norris. The journey has just begun.

BONUS

30-Days Success Challenge: Your Practical Recipe for a Healthier You.

Embark on a transformative 30-day journey towards the bdy and mind you desire with practical, daily steps designed to create lasting change. Let's break down your path to a healthier you, one day at a time.

Day 1: Goal Setting for a Healthier You
•Define your SMART weight loss goals.
•Specify the pounds or inches you want to lose, and set a realistic timeframe.

Day 2: Energizing Morning Routine
•Kickstart your metabolism with a morning workout.
•Whether it's a quick cardio session or a brisk walk, infuse your mornings with activity.

Day 3: Nutritional Audit
•Assess your current eating habits.
•Identify one unhealthy eating pattern you want to change and plan a healthier alternative.

Day 4: Connect with a Fitness Mentor
•Find a fitness influencer or expert.
•Follow their advice, routines, and use their expertise as a source of motivation.

Day 5: Master a Healthy Recipe
•Explore and master a nutritious recipe.
•Cooking your meals empowers you to control ingredients and portions.

Day 6: Gratitude for a Healthier Lifestyle
•Begin a gratitude journal focused on your health.
•Reflect on positive changes and set an optimistic tone for your weight loss journey.

Day 7: Reflect and Adjust
•Evaluate your progress.

•Adjust your goals or strategies if needed, ensuring they are realistic and achievable.

Day 8: Digital Detox for Well-being
•Declutter your digital environment.
•Unsubscribe from unhealthy food blogs, and follow nutritionists or fitness influencers.

Day 9: Expand Your Fitness Network
•Connect with like-minded individuals.
•Join online fitness communities or forums to share experiences and get support.

Day 10: Home Workout Habit
•Dedicate at least 20 minutes to a home workout.
•Choose exercises that target your weight loss goals.

Day 11: Mindful Eating Mastery
•Practice mindful eating.
•Savor each bite, eat slowly, and pay attention to hunger and fullness cues.

•Continue this weight loss journey, implementing one practical step each day. Your recipe for a healthier you is the way!
Start Your Day 1 and let the 30-day weight loss challenge redefine your path to a fitter, healthier lifestyle!

Practical Tips:
- Batch Your Tasks: Group similar tasks together to boost efficiency.
- Time Blocking: Allocate specific time blocks for crucial activities.
- Accountability Buddy: Share your goals with someone who'll keep you accountable.

Your Challenge, Your Success:
Remember, this challenge is about practical, real-world actions. Adjust the ingredients as needed. Feel free to add your own spices to make this recipe uniquely yours.
Get ready to witness the transformation. Your success story starts now. Are you up for the challenge? **Start Your Challenge and let the 30-day success recipe reshape your destiny!**

TABLE OF CONTENTS.

INTRODUCTION

What is Biohacking?

The practice of adjusting your body and mind for optimal performance is known as biohacking. It's about optimizing your biological makeup to improve your physical and mental capacities. In contrast to traditional methods, biohacking is an individual and exploratory process. It entails taking the initiative to figure out what suits you the best.

Essentially, biohacking gives you the ability to design your own wellbeing. Biohacking explores every facet of your lifestyle, from sleep and diet to exercise and cognitive function, with the aim of   maximizing   your   potential.

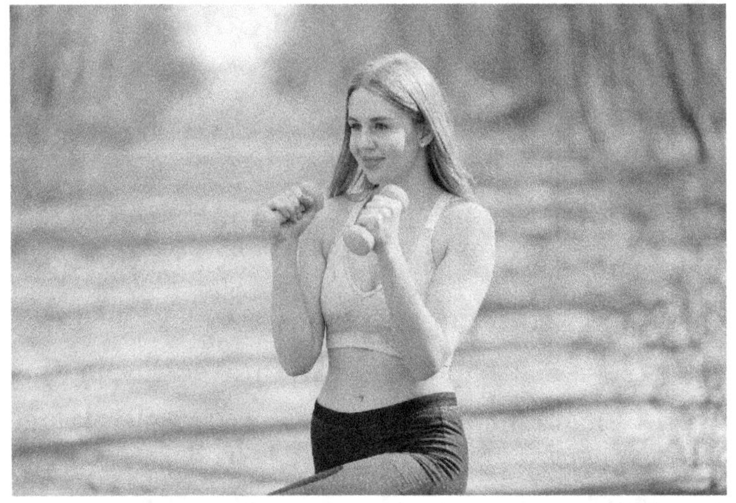

What to anticipate from the book:

This book, "Beyond Sweat and Tears: How to Acquire the Body and Mind You Desire with the Help of Bio Hackers," takes us on an enlightening journey. This book serves as your practical manual for comprehending and applying the concepts of biohacking.

Anticipate learning:

•Realistic perspectives on diet, sleep, and cognitive function via biohacking.

•Unconventional methods of staying fit that go beyond a typical gym session.

•Techniques for stress reduction, hormonal equilibrium, and fostering a positive biohacking environment.

•This book focuses on creating long-lasting habits that promote long-term well-being rather than merely offering fast cures.

So grab a seat, and let's explore the fascinating world of biohacking, where you may change your body and mind in ways you never would have imagined.

When you open "Beyond Sweat and Tears," picture this book as your ticket to a world where optimization and self-discovery are paramount. We will guide you through a series of chapters aimed at inspiring and empowering you as we reveal the mysteries of biohacking.

This book provides a toolset of options rather than a one-size-fits-all answer. Because every individual's biology is different, what works for one person may not work for another, as biohacking recognizes. You will be able to personalize your approach to biohacking and turn it into a customized journey that meets your objectives and desires with the help of useful insights, advice, and a plethora of information.

We start our trip by laying the groundwork—a way of thinking that opens up new possibilities for you. After that, we'll discuss diet, sleep, and cognitive improvement and give you practical advice on how to biohack these important aspects of your life.

However, biohacking explores the complexities of your mind and emotions in addition to the physical. Learn how to create a strong mind-body connection, regulate hormones, and handle stress. Investigate the unusual when it comes to fitness, keeping in mind that there may be paths less traveled that lead to a healthy physique.

You will come across accounts in this book of people who have used biohacking to achieve incredible metamorphoses. These stories highlight the real-world effects that biohacking may have on people's lives and function as sources of motivation.

By the time we finish our adventure, you will not only know more, but also have the know-how and insight to apply the concepts of biohacking to your everyday life. "Beyond Sweat and Tears" is more than simply a book; it's a guide to realizing your potential and living the body and mind of your dreams.

So buckle in, widen your mind, and get ready to go beyond the ordinary—into the realm of biohacking, which is really exceptional.

Chapter1.

Biohacker's Mindset - Why a Proactive Mindset Matters.

The cornerstone that sets off the thrilling world of biohacking is the Biohacker's Mindset. This chapter will open your eyes to the reasons that adopting a proactive mentality is not only advantageous but also crucial to achieving optimal health and fitness.

The Importance of a Proactive Mentality

Ownership of Your Well-Being: Having a proactive outlook means that you are taking responsibility for your health. Recognizing your ability to influence your own health is the foundation of biohacking. You are the creator of your own life when you take the initiative.

Accepting Continuous Improvement: Biohackers are aware that personal development is an ongoing endeavor. Constant improvement is the foundation of a proactive mindset. It inspires you to rise to the occasion, regard setbacks as teaching moments, and persistently look for methods to improve your mental and physical abilities.

Adaptability in the Face of Change: Your journey in biohacking is dynamic, just like life itself. Having a proactive mindset makes it easier for you to adjust to changes. Proactively adapting to the constantly changing field of health optimization, whether it is through new biohacking techniques, diet plans, or exercise regimens, guarantees that you can keep up with the times.

Self-Discovery and Experimentation: Biohacking is fundamentally an experimental field. A proactive mentality encourages you to investigate, inquire, and test out several strategies to see which ones are most effective for you. It fosters an inquisitive and introspective mindset, enabling you to customize your biohacking tactics according to your own requirements and inclinations.

Positive Effect on Motivation: Motivation is sparked by proactivity. Taking a proactive approach to biohacking increases your chances of maintaining motivation as you go. As you engage in biohacking, setting objectives, acknowledging minor accomplishments, and keeping an optimistic mindset become essential elements.

The Biohacker's Mindset essentially lays the groundwork for your metamorphosis. It matters how you go about things as much as what you do. Thus, when we dive into the upcoming chapters, remember that the proactive attitude is the cornerstone of your biohacking experience—a mindset that drives you toward a more vibrant, healthier version of yourself.

Chapter 2.

Nutrition Hacks - Simple Biohacking Nutrition Tips.

The importance of nutrition in the biohacking journey cannot be emphasized. In Chapter 2, "Nutrition Hacks," the potential of straightforward yet powerful bio-hacking techniques for enhancing your eating patterns is revealed.

Easy Bio-Hacking Dietary Advice:

1. Customized Fueling: Adjust your diet to meet your particular requirements. The first step in biohacking nutrition is figuring out what your body needs. To develop a customized feeding strategy that energizes and supports your goals,

take into account variables like metabolic rate, activity levels, and food choices.

2. Mindful Eating Habits: Biohacking involves more than just what you eat—it also involves how you eat. Accept mindful eating as a way to develop a stronger bond with your food. Enjoy every bite, eat slowly, and pay attention to your body's signals of hunger and fullness. Better nutritional absorption and digestion can result from this easy technique.

3. Intermittent Fasting: Examine the potential of this strategy for biohacking. You can optimize insulin regulation, support cellular repair, and maximize metabolic performance by adding deliberate fasting periods. Discover how to incorporate intermittent fasting into your daily routine for improved mental and physical health.

4. Nutrient-Dense Superfoods: Eat foods high in nutrients to enhance your diet. Foods high in antioxidants, vitamins, and minerals are given priority by biohackers. Learn about a range of

superfoods that can improve your dietary intake and promote general health and wellbeing.

5. Hydration Optimization: One of the main biohacking techniques is staying hydrated. Investigate ways to maximize your water intake while taking electrolyte balance and water quality into account. Sufficient hydration is essential for optimal cellular health, energy production, and cognitive performance.

6. Strategic Supplementation: Increase the amount of nutrients you consume by strategically adding supplements. Supplements can help biohackers make up for any nutritional inadequacies in their diet. Find out about essential supplements, such omega-3 fatty acids, vitamin D, and adaptogens, that can help you on your biohacking path.

7. Biohacking Your Gut: Learn about the state of your digestive system. The goal of biohacking your gut is to cultivate a diversified and well-balanced microbiota. Discover how to

include fermented foods, probiotics, and prebiotics in your diet to support gut health, which affects both mental and physical wellness.

Your road map for negotiating the complex terrain of biohacking diet is provided in Chapter 2. With the help of these straightforward but effective suggestions, you can change the way you feel about food and use it as a valuable ally to achieve your goals of peak performance and wellness. When you go out on this nutritional biohacking adventure, keep in mind that minor adjustments can have a big impact.

Beyond sweat and tears

Chapter 3.

Sleep and Recovery - Improving Sleep for Better Health.

In Chapter 3, "Sleep and Recovery," the biohacker's pursuit of optimal well-being places a strong emphasis on the sometimes underappreciated topic of sleep. Learn how developing the skill of rest can significantly improve mental clarity, physical vigor, and general health.

Increasing Sleep Quality to Boost Health:

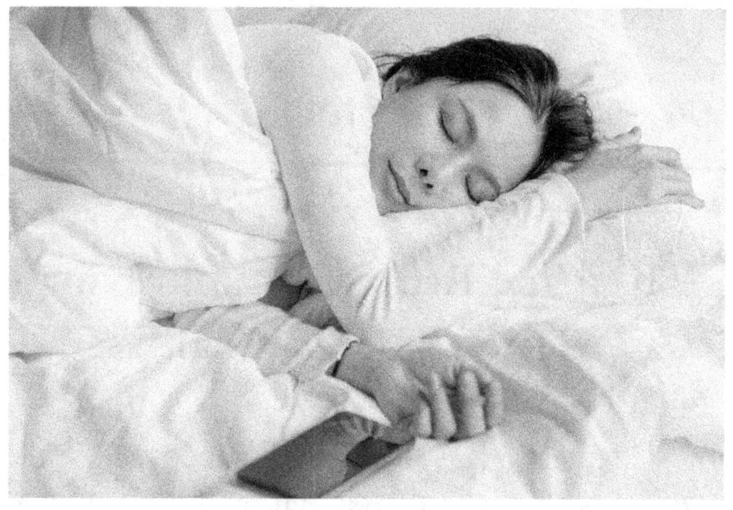

1.Recognizing Sleep Cycles: By being aware of your sleep's inherent cycles, you can biohack it. Examine the two types of sleep—REM and non-REM—and how each affects cognitive and physical recovery. Discover how to lengthen your sleep to best suit your needs.

2. Establishing a Sleep Sanctuary: Make your bedroom a restful retreat. Learn biohacking techniques to create the ideal sleeping environment, taking into account factors like temperature, lighting, and reducing technology

distractions. A sleep sanctuary encourages deeper, more revitalizing sleep.

3. Routines and Rituals for Bedtime: Create a biohacking nighttime ritual. Examine the significance of regular sleep schedules and relaxing routines before to going to bed. Try some relaxation methods to tell your body when it's time to relax, including meditation or light stretching.

4. Digital Detox Before Bed: Adopt a digital detox to biohack your evenings. Examine how screens affect the quality of your sleep and learn how to reduce artificial light exposure before bed. Discover how to establish a technology-free bedtime routine to enhance your quality of sleep.

5. Nutrition to Promote Sleep: Learn how diet and sleep are related. Use diet biohacking to incorporate foods and drinks that help you fall asleep. Examine the advantages of foods high in magnesium, herbal teas, and snacks that promote calm and help you get a better night's sleep.

6. Circadian Rhythms and Chronobiology:
Explore the field of chronobiology. Recognize the effects of circadian rhythms on your body's internal clock and how it affects wakefulness and sleep. To get better sleep, biohack your daily schedule to match your circadian cycle.

7. Biohacking Power Naps: Discover how taking deliberate naps can help you feel refreshed. Find out how taking deliberate, brief naps might improve your happiness, alertness, and cognitive function. Learn how to take power naps without disturbing your sleep at night.

8. Recuperation Strategies: Optimize your recuperation in both awake and slumbering phases. Examine the benefits of massage, relaxation techniques, and other recovery methods for promoting the best possible physical and mental healing. Recognize the benefits of getting enough sleep for daytime recuperation.

Your in-depth manual for biohacking the cycle of sleep and recuperation can be found in Chapter 3. By putting these techniques into practice, you'll improve both the amount and quality of your sleep, which will have a positive impact on your general health and wellbeing. As you explore the realm of sleep optimization, keep in mind that the cornerstone of your biohacking adventure is a physically and mentally rested body.

Chapter 4.

Cognitive Boosts - Unleashing the Power of Your Mind.

Salutations to all other biohackers! This chapter is crucial as we go deeply into the intriguing field of "Cognitive Boosts: Bio-hacks for a Sharper Mind." Get ready to go on an adventure that will maximize your mental capabilities and improve your ability to think clearly, concentrate, and perform cognitively.

Developing Your Mind's Potential:

Introducing Nootropics and Smart Supplements: An introduction to the realm of cognitive boosters. Learn about the biohacker's toolkit of intelligent supplements and nootropics that can improve mental performance. Discover how these medications, which range from natural ingredients to well developed formulas, might improve your cognitive ability.

1 Exercises for Brain Training: Take part in activities that make your brain muscles contract. Using brain-training methods to improve memory, problem-solving abilities, and general cognitive agility is known as "biohacking" cognition. Play games, solve puzzles, and engage in mindfulness exercises to maintain mental sharpness.

2.Practices for Mindful Meditation: Explore the transforming potential of mindfulness. Practice attentive meditation to biohack your mental clarity. Discover how meditation improves focus, attention, and the capacity to handle the challenges of daily life with clarity in addition to lowering stress.

3. Cognitive Load Management: Improving your brain's information processing capacity is a key

component of biohacking your cognitive load. Examine methods for organizing and prioritizing work, clearing your mind, and making decisions more quickly. To maintain mental clarity over time, learn how to prevent cognitive overload.

4. Get Good Sleep for Cognitive Renewal: Understand how sleep and cognitive function are mutually dependent. Explore the science behind how sleep aids in the consolidation of memories, the solution of problems, and creative thought. Use biohacks to enhance the quality of your sleep to accelerate cognitive regeneration.

Investigate the Cognitive Advantages of Intermittent Fasting for Brain Health. By biohacking your dietary habits, you can improve attention, clarity, and neuroplasticity in addition to other aspects of brain function. Find out how improved cognitive function and fasting are related.

5. Hydration and Brain Function: Hydration is important for cognitive biohacking, not just for

the physical body. Find out how drinking enough water helps the brain work at its best, impacting mood, focus, and information processing. Learn how to make sure your brain is getting the moisture it requires.

6. Utilizing biohacking: Accept the idea of neuroplasticity, or the capacity of your brain to change and restructure. You can biohack the wiring of your brain by doing things that cause neuroplastic alterations. Develop your cognitive flexibility by taking on new challenges and expanding your mind's horizons.

Your manual for improving your mental game is in Chapter 4. You will strengthen your cognitive resilience and improve your mental acuity by putting these biohacks into practice.
Recall that your brain is a dynamic, flexible powerhouse that you can fully utilize with the correct biohacking techniques. Get ready to see your mind's amazing powers come to life as you set off on this cognitive enhancement trip

Chapter 5:

Unconventional Fitness - Redefining Your Journey to Wellness

Salutations, exercise aficionados! You're invited to embrace "Unconventional Fitness: Different Approaches to Staying Fit" and reject conventional thinking in Chapter 5. Prepare to discover cutting-edge and practical methods for toning your body, boosting your vitality, and completely changing how you maintain optimal physical health.

1.Redefining Your Health-Related Journey:

•Beyond the Conventional Gym Workout: Go beyond the limitations of the standard gym regimen. The concept of unconventional fitness questions the status quo and motivates you to look into different types of exercise that suit your requirements and interests. Say goodbye to boredom and hello to a wide variety of activities that turn remaining in shape into a thrilling journey.

Rekindle your love of movement with a functional movement training program. Exercises that are more akin to everyday activities are prioritized in unconventional fitness, which improves your general strength, flexibility, and coordination. For a body that functions at its best and seems fit, learn how to incorporate functional exercises into your program.

Unleash the power of your own body with bodyweight mastery. Explore the world of bodyweight workouts that provide amazing results without the need for expensive equipment. Learn how developing your calisthenics skills can help you develop functional strength, sculpt your body, and enhance your agility.

•Outdoor Adventures as Exercise: Take your workout outside and break free from the walls. Accepting nature as your personal exercise facility is encouraged by unconventional fitness. Discover how the great outdoors may enhance the advantages of your fitness journey, whether you choose to hike, trail run, or participate in outdoor sports.

•Practices for Mind-Body Fusion: Investigate methods of physical fitness that go beyond it. Unconventional fitness acknowledges the close relationship between the body and mind. Take up exercises like yoga, Pilates, or martial arts to build mental toughness and mindfulness in addition to strengthening your body.

2.Variations in High-Intensity Interval Training (HIIT):

Increase your level of fitness with effective and energetic exercises. Unconventional HIIT variations combine short bursts of high-intensity activity with rest intervals or lower-intensity activities to give your regimen an exciting twist. Enjoy a variety of fun training methods while reaping the time-saving advantages of HIIT.

Using dance and movement therapies, you may make your exercise regimen a joyful dance. Dance and movement therapy are examples of unconventional fitness. Find out how dancing exercises increase your heart health as well as your rhythm, coordination, and overall enjoyment of being active.

•Adventuresome Fitness Challenges: Accept and rise to the occasion when it comes to fitness. You're invited to take part in fitness challenges and daring activities that stretch your boundaries while you pursue unconventional fitness. Get the rush of pushing yourself to new limits in your fitness journey, whether it is through obstacle courses or adventure events.

Your pass to an extraordinary fitness adventure is provided by Chapter 5. Adopting non-traditional methods will help you stay in shape while also bringing you delight and excitement.

Get ready to rethink what exercise means to you and explore a universe of options that can accommodate your own tastes and goals. Remember this as you go into this unorthodox world of fitness: the best workout is the one you look forward to!

Chapter 6.

Hormonal Balance - Harmonizing the Symphony Within.

Hi there, those that love health! In Chapter 6, you are invited to explore the complex realm of "Hormonal Balance: Understanding and Optimizing Hormones," on a voyage deep within your body. Prepare to explore the hormone symphony that plays a role in many facets of your health and learn how to adjust it to get your best possible health.

Calming the Internal Symphony:

Think of your hormones as messengers, delivering important information to each and every cell in your body. We examine the major actors in this chapter, including insulin, cortisol, estrogen, testosterone, and more. The first step to balancing the complex dance of hormones is to understand their roles.

•Hormones' Effect on Body Composition:
Examine the enormous effect hormones have on the composition of your body. Hormonal balance is crucial whether your goal is fat loss or muscle building. Discover how to achieve your exercise objectives and shape your body by optimizing your hormonal environment.

•The Function of Nutrition in Hormonal Balance:
Your hormonal symphony is powerfully conducted by the food you eat. Learn how dietary decisions affect the balance and production of hormones. Discover how to create a diet that promotes hormonal balance and general well-being, from macronutrient ratios to foods high in micronutrients.

•Physical Activity and Hormonal Optimization:
Exercise is a conductor of hormonal homeostasis

in addition to being a means of burning calories. Learn how various forms of exercise affect hormones, from the mood-boosting properties of cardio to the anabolic effects of strength training. Adapt your workout regimen to maximize your hormones.

•Control and Management of Stress: Get to know cortisol, the hormone that causes stress, and discover how to get along with it. Learn how the delicate balance between relaxation and stress affects hormone homeostasis. Learn useful techniques for stress management and cortisol regulation for general hormonal health.

The Impact of Sleep on Hormonal Health
Your nightly ritual is a nocturnal hormonal harmony conductor. Explore the relationship between sleep and hormones to learn how the type and length of your sleep affect hormones that control your appetite and growth hormone production.

Discover the complex dance between estrogen and testosterone in "Balancing Sex Hormones." When it comes to sex hormones, hormonal balance is especially important because it affects fertility, mood, and energy levels. Discover how a balanced lifestyle, proper diet, and mindfulness all lead to harmony.

Hormone Optimization via Biohacking: A Guide to Hormone Health Biohacking. Learn cutting-edge tactics and biohacks to take control of your hormonal orchestra. Find out how to biohack hormone balance through targeted supplements and intermittent fasting.

Your manual for deciphering the inner symphony and adjusting your hormone balance for optimum health is Chapter 6. You can create a bright and balanced life in addition to balancing your internal symphony by learning about the role of hormones and applying biohacking techniques.

Beyond sweat and tears

Chapter 7.

Stress Management - Nurturing Your Inner Sanctuary.

Greetings and welcome to Chapter 7, in which we delve into the art of "Stress Management: Bio-hacks for Stress Relief." This chapter delves into the busy terrain of your everyday existence, revealing practical biohacks to reduce stress and create a peaceful inner haven.

Taking Care of Your Inner Refuge:

Recognizing the Stress Response: Think of stress as your body's alarm system, alerting you to potential dangers. This chapter begins with an exploration of the complexities of the stress response, illuminating the physiological and psychological transformations that take place when stress becomes a problem.

Stress Reduction and Mindfulness: Learn about mindfulness, a potent tool for managing stress. Examine useful methods to help you stay in the present, such deep breathing and meditation. Find out how these techniques help retrain your brain to become resilient and calm.

Nutrition's Effect on Stress:
Explore the world of dietary tactics to strengthen your ability to cope with stress. Learn how specific meals and dietary decisions can affect neurotransmitters and stress hormones, giving your body the energy it needs to overcome obstacles in life.

Adaptogens and Stress Resilience: Get to know adaptogens, the gifts of nature that reduce stress. Discover how to help your body adjust to stress with the help of these herbal companions. Find out how adaptogens, such as rhodiola and ashwagandha, can improve your ability to withstand stress and support general wellbeing.

Physical Activity as Stress Reduction: It turns out that exercise is a really effective biohack for reducing stress. Explore the link between exercise and lowering stress levels and how movement releases endorphins, which are your body's natural mood enhancers. Customize your exercise regimen to reap the greatest benefits in reducing stress.

Establishing a Stress-Resilient Setting:
Your environment is crucial for managing stress. Make adjustments to your surroundings that promote calmness to biohack your area. Some examples of these adjustments include clearing out clutter, adding calming hues, or including more natural elements into your everyday routine.

Stress-Reduction Mind-Body Techniques: Give yourself over to mind-body techniques that are meant to reduce stress. Learn how these techniques, which range from progressive muscle relaxation to guided visualization, balance your mental and physical states and help you create a calm haven in the middle of life's stresses.

Digital wellness and technology detoxification: unplug to refuel. Rethink how you interact with technology by acknowledging how it affects your stress levels. Examine methods for going digital-free and setting limits to make time for rest and renewal.

Your guide to creating an inner sanctuary amidst the chaos of life is found in Chapter 7. By implementing these biohacks for stress management, you'll not only be able to overcome obstacles more easily but also develop a strong, calm mindset. Now, let's set off on this trip of stress management and self-care, where serenity becomes your constant traveling companion on the road to wellbeing.

Chapter 8.

Mind-Body Connection.

- How mental and physical health are connected.

Salutations to all my fellow vitality explorers! Chapter 8 takes us on a deep dive into the complex interactions of "Mind-Body Connection: How Mental and Physical Health Are Connected." Get ready to see how your ideas, feelings, and physical health work together to reveal the mysteries of holistic health.

Crossing the Well-Being Gulf:

The Symbiotic Dance: Picture your body and mind dancing together gracefully as partners. We'll look at the mutually beneficial relationship between mental and physical health in this chapter. Explore how your body, mind, and emotions work together to create your overall level of well-being.

Effect of Thoughts on Physiology: Behold the ability of your thoughts to change you. Recognize how your mental environment affects the physiological reactions in your body. Learn how to think positively to improve your physical well-being while thinking negatively or under stress might have the opposite effect.

Emotions as Messengers: Your inner world is communicated through your emotions. Examine the ways in which your body communicates with your emotions, both happy and difficult. Acquire the ability to decipher these signals and channel emotional energy towards a more harmonious mind-body relationship.

Stress, Cortisol, and Physical Health: In the mind-body link, stress is a major factor. Discover how stress affects cortisol release and how that affects physical health. Learn biohacks to help you reduce stress and encourage a better mental-physical balance.

Harmony-Focusing Mind-Body Techniques: Engage in mind-body techniques that promote harmony. These practices, which span the spectrum from mindful movement to tai chi and yoga, integrate mental and physical well-being. Feel the transformation that occurs when your thoughts are in harmony with deliberate movement.

Explore the intriguing realm of the gut-brain axis on this journey. Examine the relationship between your gut's health and your mental well-being. Learn the significant relationship that exists between mood, general well-being, and intestinal health.

Psychosomatic Impact on Health: Observe the impact of psychosomatic factors on one's health. Examine the ways that psychological issues might cause physical problems. Learn how to heal psychosomatic imbalances and foster a more balanced relationship between your mind and body.

Developing Positive Mindsets: Make use of optimism's power. Find out how having a happy outlook on life might affect your physical well-being. Examine doable strategies to promote resilience, optimism, and a positive view on life.

Your manual for deciphering the complex conversation between your body and mind is Chapter 8. Acknowledging the significant relationship between mental and physical well-being will set you on the path to achieving holistic wellbeing.

Now, let's investigate this fusion of the mind and body, in which every feeling and idea turns into a brushstroke on the picture of your colorful, interwoven life. Welcome to the world where the body and mind work together to create a masterpiece of harmony and life.

Chapter 9.

Environment Matters - Crafting the Canvas of Well-being.

Greetings, wellness architects! Chapter 9, "Environment Matters: Creating a Supportive Bio-hacking Environment," invites us to investigate the significant impact of our environment. This chapter will reveal the transforming impact of creating a well-being sanctuary by arranging your surroundings to align with your biohacking objectives.

Creating the Well-Being Canvas:

The Environmental Symphony: Visualize your surroundings as the orchestra directing your biohacking endeavors. We'll explore the ways that your physical environment—at home and at work—affects your emotional and physical well-being. Discover the skill of creating a space that supports your health.

Observe the enchantment of decluttering to gain mental clarity. Learn how mental clarity and focus can be enhanced by a neat physical environment. By adopting minimalism and order, you can biohack your surroundings and create a setting that enhances your mental and emotional health.

Natural Components for Calm: Calm is largely found in nature. Investigate biohacking by introducing natural ingredients into your surroundings. Find out how adding plants, making the most of natural light, or including water features may help create a peaceful, revitalizing space.

Technology Optimization for Balance: Take care when navigating the digital world. Use technology biohacking to find a balance between connectedness and peace of mind. Discover how to make the most of your digital surroundings, improve concentration, and make time for rest and renewal in a world where connectivity is growing.

Soundscapes for Wellness: Harness the restorative properties of sound. Learn how soundscapes, such as nature sounds and relaxing music, can affect your stress levels and mood.

By biohacking your aural environment, you may establish a peaceful background that upholds your emotional and mental balance.

Ergonomics for Physical Health: The physical surroundings you live in have an impact on your health. Examine ergonomics concepts to biohack your living and working environments. Optimize your physical surroundings for improved well-being, from furniture alignment to the creation of spaces that encourage activity.

Social Connection in Your Space: You may create social ties in your space. Learn how your environment's layout and design affect social interactions. By biohacking your environment, you can improve your emotional and mental health by fostering relationships with friends, family, and the community.

Establishing Routines and Rituals: Your daily landscape is shaped by your routines and rituals. Examine the possibilities for biohacking with deliberate everyday routines. Discover how creating supporting rituals can influence your general well-being, from nighttime routines that encourage peaceful sleep to morning rituals that establish a pleasant tone.

Chapter 10.

Long-Term Bio-hacking - Sustaining the Flame of Well-being.

Hi there, In Chapter 10, we are invited to delve into the practice of "Long-Term Biohacking: Incorporating Bio-hacks for a Lasting Lifestyle." We'll navigate the landscape of sustainable well-being in this chapter, so your journey to biohacking is a transforming, lifetime marathon rather than a quick fix.

Maintaining the Wellness Flame:

The Key to Extended Biohacking:
Long-term biohacking is a dedication to long-term well-being rather than a search for short-term solutions. We'll get into the fundamentals of developing long-lasting routines and habits, so that your journey toward

biohacking becomes an essential aspect of your life.

Accept the Power of Progressive Goal Setting: Make the most of this approach. By acknowledging that sustained change happens in small, manageable increments, you can biohack your goal-setting process. Discover how to celebrate little triumphs and set goals to generate a sense of accomplishment that will motivate long-term dedication.

Adaptability and Evolution: The voyage of the biohacker is a dynamic undertaking. Discover the skill of adaptation, understanding that you may need to make changes to your biohacking routine over time. Develop the ability to pay attention to your body and mind so that you can make decisions based on what your needs and goals are right now.

Conscious Nutrition as a Lifestyle: Eating well is a lifetime commitment; it's not a quick fix. Make mindful eating a way of life to biohack your relationship with food. As you embark on an enduring path of well-being, learn about the concepts of intuitive eating, balanced nutrition, and the delight of savoring each meal.

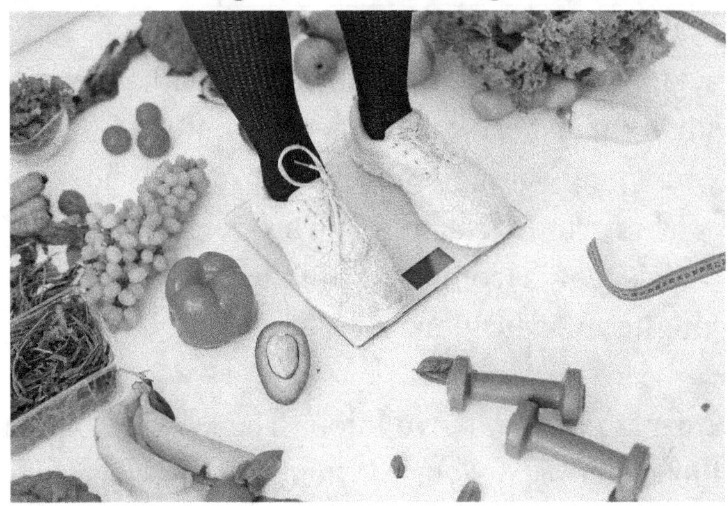

Including Play and Joy: Play and joy foster a state of well-being. Discover how adding things that actually make you happy can biohack your life. Engage in enjoyable activities, hobbies, or artistic endeavors to bring happiness into your life and make sure that happiness is a journey rather than a destination.

Communities and Support Systems: In a community that is supportive, long-term well-being is fostered. By cultivating relationships that support your health objectives, you can biohack your social networks. Join or start networks with like-minded people who can support you and offer advice based on your experiences biohacking.

Integration of the Mind and Body as a Lifestyle: The mind-body connection is a way of life, not just a passing trend. Examine how your everyday life is weaved together with mind-body practices. Make these activities a seamless part of your daily, from mindful movement to meditation, to support long-term overall well-being.

Introspection and Ongoing Education: Prolonged biohackers are lifelong learners. Examine the practice of introspection and lifelong learning, understanding that happiness is a constant process of self-exploration. Develop an inquisitive and receptive attitude toward novel biohacking techniques that correspond with your developing health comprehension.

We close the gap between short-term biohacking gains and long-term lifestyle maintenance for holistic well-being in these last chapters. As you adopt the practices of long-term bio-hacking and environment optimization, keep in mind that maintaining your health is an ongoing journey, with each biohack serving as a brushstroke that adds to the masterpiece that is your robust and colorful life. Cheers to biohacking!

Conclusion.

Recap and encouragement for a biohacking journey.

Greetings, fellow biohackers

My sincere congrats on starting this path of biohacking as we get to the finish of this life-changing adventure through the world of wellbeing. You've studied the complex web of your own health, investigated the relationships between the body and mind, and adopted a variety of biohacks to design a vibrant life.

A Summary of Our Biohacking Journey:

We've read through chapters together that have revealed the best ways to eat, the value of getting restful sleep, techniques to improve cognitive function, and the skill of creating an environment that promotes wellbeing. Every chapter has served as a stepping stone on your journey to wellbeing, covering topics like stress management, hormonal balance, the mind-body connection, and the timeless principles of long-term biohacking.

We've explored your inner haven and come to understand the mental benefits of clear spaces and natural elements. We now know about the intricate relationship between gut health and mood, the calming effects of mindful activities, and the dance between ideas and physiology. Our investigation went beyond the individual, highlighting the value of a nurturing environment and environmentally friendly lifestyle options.

Motivation for the Journey Ahead:
I want to encourage you as you stand on the brink of your continued journey into biohacking. Recall that biohacking is an ongoing journey rather than a destination—a dynamic dance with your unique vitality. Accept the lessons you've learned and incorporate them into your everyday activities.

Honor Your Progress Rather Than Perfection: Each little step you've taken is a victory. Celebrate your accomplishments since long-lasting transformation is the result of repeated efforts. Understand that the process of self-discovery that is biohacking is a success with every discovery.

Pay Attention to Your Body and Mind: These are your guides. Pay close attention, tune in, and modify your biohacking tactics as necessary. Accept the ups and downs of your trip and the fact that it's normal for your requirements to change over time.

Adopt a Holistic Perspective: A holistic approach considers all aspects of your life. Keep incorporating biohacks into your everyday routine to promote a healthy lifestyle that feeds your body, mind, and spirit.

Become a Part of a Community: Talk to others who share your interests about your adventure. Develop relationships with other biohackers in the community by sharing knowledge and words of support. A network of support can serve as a guiding light in both difficult and joyful times.

Develop a Curious Mindset: The field of biohacking is one of ongoing exploration. Have an inquisitive attitude and be receptive to new findings, methods, and tools that support your objectives. Continue to be involved and relish the process of discovering your own abilities.

Treat yourself with kindness: achieving well-being is a journey, not a sprint. Recognize that obstacles are a part of the path and treat yourself with kindness. Recognize that every day offers the possibility of rejuvenation and approach obstacles with fortitude and compassion for oneself.

Finally, I want to thank you for making an investment in your health and wellbeing. I hope that your road towards biohacking brings you happiness, perseverance, and constant improvement.

Remember that the best biohack is the one that gets you closer to the healthy, robust, and contented version of yourself as you explore the unexplored regions of your own vitality.

With wellness wishes,
[Catherine.J.Norris]

Your Review Matters:
If you've had the pleasure of diving into [Beyond Sweat and Tears], we invite you to share your thoughts. Your reviews contribute to the tapestry of experiences, helping others discover the transformative power within these pages. Join the conversation and let your voice be heard!